Tennis Nutrition Log and Diary

This Book Belongs To:

_____

Visit http://elegantnotebooks.com for more sports training books.

Training Log and Diary
Nutrition Log and Diary
Strength and Conditioning Log and Diary

DATE:	WEEK:	WEIGHT:

BREAKFAST	Protein	Carbs	Fat	Fiber	Sodium	Calories

SNACK	Protein	Carbs	Fat	Fiber	Sodium	Calories

LUNCH	Protein	Carbs	Fat	Fiber	Sodium	Calories

SNACK	Protein	Carbs	Fat	Fiber	Sodium	Calories

DINNER	Protein	Carbs	Fat	Fiber	Sodium	Calories

SNACK	Protein	Carbs	Fat	Fiber	Sodium	Calories

DAILY TOTALS						
DAILY GOALS						
% DAILY GOALS	%	%	%	%	%	%

WATER   1 cup per circle
(1 cup = 8 ounces ~ 240ml)   ○○○○○○○○○○○○○○○○

DATE: _____ **WEEK:** _____ **WEIGHT:** _____

BREAKFAST	Protein	Carbs	Fat	Fiber	Sodium	Calories

SNACK	Protein	Carbs	Fat	Fiber	Sodium	Calories

LUNCH	Protein	Carbs	Fat	Fiber	Sodium	Calories

SNACK	Protein	Carbs	Fat	Fiber	Sodium	Calories

DINNER	Protein	Carbs	Fat	Fiber	Sodium	Calories

SNACK	Protein	Carbs	Fat	Fiber	Sodium	Calories

DAILY TOTALS						
DAILY GOALS						
% DAILY GOALS	%	%	%	%	%	%

WATER   1 cup per circle
(1 cup = 8 ounces ~ 240ml)   ○ ○ ○ ○ ○ ○ ○ ○ ○ ○ ○ ○ ○ ○ ○ ○

DATE: _____ **WEEK:** _____ **WEIGHT:** _____

BREAKFAST	Protein	Carbs	Fat	Fiber	Sodium	Calories

SNACK	Protein	Carbs	Fat	Fiber	Sodium	Calories

LUNCH	Protein	Carbs	Fat	Fiber	Sodium	Calories

SNACK	Protein	Carbs	Fat	Fiber	Sodium	Calories

DINNER	Protein	Carbs	Fat	Fiber	Sodium	Calories

SNACK	Protein	Carbs	Fat	Fiber	Sodium	Calories

DAILY TOTALS						
DAILY GOALS						
% DAILY GOALS	%	%	%	%	%	%

WATER 1 cup per circle
(1 cup = 8 ounces ~ 240ml)

○ ○ ○ ○ ○ ○ ○ ○ ○ ○ ○ ○ ○ ○ ○ ○ ○

DATE: _____ **WEEK:** _____ **WEIGHT:** _____

BREAKFAST	Protein	Carbs	Fat	Fiber	Sodium	Calories

SNACK	Protein	Carbs	Fat	Fiber	Sodium	Calories

LUNCH	Protein	Carbs	Fat	Fiber	Sodium	Calories

SNACK	Protein	Carbs	Fat	Fiber	Sodium	Calories

DINNER	Protein	Carbs	Fat	Fiber	Sodium	Calories

SNACK	Protein	Carbs	Fat	Fiber	Sodium	Calories

DAILY TOTALS						
DAILY GOALS						
% DAILY GOALS	%	%	%	%	%	%

WATER 1 cup per circle
(1 cup = 8 ounces ~ 240ml)   ○ ○ ○ ○ ○ ○ ○ ○ ○ ○ ○ ○ ○ ○ ○ ○

DATE: _____ **WEEK:** _____ **WEIGHT:** _____

BREAKFAST	Protein	Carbs	Fat	Fiber	Sodium	Calories

SNACK	Protein	Carbs	Fat	Fiber	Sodium	Calories

LUNCH	Protein	Carbs	Fat	Fiber	Sodium	Calories

SNACK	Protein	Carbs	Fat	Fiber	Sodium	Calories

DINNER	Protein	Carbs	Fat	Fiber	Sodium	Calories

SNACK	Protein	Carbs	Fat	Fiber	Sodium	Calories

DAILY TOTALS						
DAILY GOALS						
% DAILY GOALS	%	%	%	%	%	%

WATER   1 cup per circle
(1 cup = 8 ounces ~ 240ml)   ◯ ◯ ◯ ◯ ◯ ◯ ◯ ◯ ◯ ◯ ◯ ◯ ◯ ◯

DATE: _____ **WEEK:** _____ **WEIGHT:** _____

BREAKFAST	Protein	Carbs	Fat	Fiber	Sodium	Calories

SNACK	Protein	Carbs	Fat	Fiber	Sodium	Calories

LUNCH	Protein	Carbs	Fat	Fiber	Sodium	Calories

SNACK	Protein	Carbs	Fat	Fiber	Sodium	Calories

DINNER	Protein	Carbs	Fat	Fiber	Sodium	Calories

SNACK	Protein	Carbs	Fat	Fiber	Sodium	Calories

DAILY TOTALS						
DAILY GOALS						
% DAILY GOALS	%	%	%	%	%	%

WATER   1 cup per circle
(1 cup = 8 ounces ~ 240ml)   ◯ ◯ ◯ ◯ ◯ ◯ ◯ ◯ ◯ ◯ ◯ ◯ ◯ ◯

DATE:		WEEK:		WEIGHT:			

BREAKFAST	Protein	Carbs	Fat	Fiber	Sodium	Calories

SNACK	Protein	Carbs	Fat	Fiber	Sodium	Calories

LUNCH	Protein	Carbs	Fat	Fiber	Sodium	Calories

SNACK	Protein	Carbs	Fat	Fiber	Sodium	Calories

DINNER	Protein	Carbs	Fat	Fiber	Sodium	Calories

SNACK	Protein	Carbs	Fat	Fiber	Sodium	Calories

DAILY TOTALS						
DAILY GOALS						
% DAILY GOALS	%	%	%	%	%	%

WATER   1 cup per circle
(1 cup = 8 ounces ~ 240ml)   ○ ○ ○ ○ ○ ○ ○ ○ ○ ○ ○ ○ ○ ○

DATE: _____ **WEEK:** _____ **WEIGHT:** _____

BREAKFAST	Protein	Carbs	Fat	Fiber	Sodium	Calories

SNACK	Protein	Carbs	Fat	Fiber	Sodium	Calories

LUNCH	Protein	Carbs	Fat	Fiber	Sodium	Calories

SNACK	Protein	Carbs	Fat	Fiber	Sodium	Calories

DINNER	Protein	Carbs	Fat	Fiber	Sodium	Calories

SNACK	Protein	Carbs	Fat	Fiber	Sodium	Calories

DAILY TOTALS						
DAILY GOALS						
% DAILY GOALS	%	%	%	%	%	%

WATER   1 cup per circle
(1 cup = 8 ounces ~ 240ml)   ○ ○ ○ ○ ○ ○ ○ ○ ○ ○ ○ ○ ○ ○ ○ ○

DATE:	WEEK:	WEIGHT:

BREAKFAST	Protein	Carbs	Fat	Fiber	Sodium	Calories
SNACK	Protein	Carbs	Fat	Fiber	Sodium	Calories
LUNCH	Protein	Carbs	Fat	Fiber	Sodium	Calories
SNACK	Protein	Carbs	Fat	Fiber	Sodium	Calories
DINNER	Protein	Carbs	Fat	Fiber	Sodium	Calories
SNACK	Protein	Carbs	Fat	Fiber	Sodium	Calories
DAILY TOTALS						
DAILY GOALS						
% DAILY GOALS	%	%	%	%	%	%

WATER   1 cup per circle
(1 cup = 8 ounces ~ 240ml)   ○○○○○○○○○○○○○○○○

DATE: _____   **WEEK:** _____   **WEIGHT:** _____

BREAKFAST	Protein	Carbs	Fat	Fiber	Sodium	Calories

SNACK	Protein	Carbs	Fat	Fiber	Sodium	Calories

LUNCH	Protein	Carbs	Fat	Fiber	Sodium	Calories

SNACK	Protein	Carbs	Fat	Fiber	Sodium	Calories

DINNER	Protein	Carbs	Fat	Fiber	Sodium	Calories

SNACK	Protein	Carbs	Fat	Fiber	Sodium	Calories

DAILY TOTALS						
DAILY GOALS						
% DAILY GOALS	%	%	%	%	%	%

WATER   1 cup per circle
(1 cup = 8 ounces ~ 240ml)   ○○○○○○○○○○○○○○○○

DATE: _____   **WEEK:** _____   **WEIGHT:** _____

BREAKFAST	Protein	Carbs	Fat	Fiber	Sodium	Calories

SNACK	Protein	Carbs	Fat	Fiber	Sodium	Calories

LUNCH	Protein	Carbs	Fat	Fiber	Sodium	Calories

SNACK	Protein	Carbs	Fat	Fiber	Sodium	Calories

DINNER	Protein	Carbs	Fat	Fiber	Sodium	Calories

SNACK	Protein	Carbs	Fat	Fiber	Sodium	Calories

DAILY TOTALS						
DAILY GOALS						
% DAILY GOALS	%	%	%	%	%	%

WATER   1 cup per circle
(1 cup = 8 ounces ~ 240ml)   ○ ○ ○ ○ ○ ○ ○ ○ ○ ○ ○ ○ ○ ○ ○

DATE:	WEEK:	WEIGHT:

BREAKFAST	Protein	Carbs	Fat	Fiber	Sodium	Calories

SNACK	Protein	Carbs	Fat	Fiber	Sodium	Calories

LUNCH	Protein	Carbs	Fat	Fiber	Sodium	Calories

SNACK	Protein	Carbs	Fat	Fiber	Sodium	Calories

DINNER	Protein	Carbs	Fat	Fiber	Sodium	Calories

SNACK	Protein	Carbs	Fat	Fiber	Sodium	Calories

DAILY TOTALS						
DAILY GOALS						
% DAILY GOALS	%	%	%	%	%	%

WATER   1 cup per circle
(1 cup = 8 ounces ~ 240ml)   ○ ○ ○ ○ ○ ○ ○ ○ ○ ○ ○ ○ ○ ○ ○ ○

DATE: _____ **WEEK:** _____ **WEIGHT:** _____

BREAKFAST	Protein	Carbs	Fat	Fiber	Sodium	Calories

SNACK	Protein	Carbs	Fat	Fiber	Sodium	Calories

LUNCH	Protein	Carbs	Fat	Fiber	Sodium	Calories

SNACK	Protein	Carbs	Fat	Fiber	Sodium	Calories

DINNER	Protein	Carbs	Fat	Fiber	Sodium	Calories

SNACK	Protein	Carbs	Fat	Fiber	Sodium	Calories
DAILY TOTALS						
DAILY GOALS						
% DAILY GOALS	%	%	%	%	%	%

WATER 1 cup per circle
(1 cup = 8 ounces ~ 240ml) ◯◯◯◯◯◯◯◯◯◯◯◯◯◯◯◯

DATE: _____ **WEEK:** _____ **WEIGHT:** _____

BREAKFAST	Protein	Carbs	Fat	Fiber	Sodium	Calories

SNACK	Protein	Carbs	Fat	Fiber	Sodium	Calories

LUNCH	Protein	Carbs	Fat	Fiber	Sodium	Calories

SNACK	Protein	Carbs	Fat	Fiber	Sodium	Calories

DINNER	Protein	Carbs	Fat	Fiber	Sodium	Calories

SNACK	Protein	Carbs	Fat	Fiber	Sodium	Calories

DAILY TOTALS						
DAILY GOALS						
% DAILY GOALS	%	%	%	%	%	%

WATER 1 cup per circle
(1 cup = 8 ounces ~ 240ml)   ○○○○○○○○○○○○○○○○○○○

DATE: _____ **WEEK:** _____ **WEIGHT:** _____

BREAKFAST	Protein	Carbs	Fat	Fiber	Sodium	Calories

SNACK	Protein	Carbs	Fat	Fiber	Sodium	Calories

LUNCH	Protein	Carbs	Fat	Fiber	Sodium	Calories

SNACK	Protein	Carbs	Fat	Fiber	Sodium	Calories

DINNER	Protein	Carbs	Fat	Fiber	Sodium	Calories

SNACK	Protein	Carbs	Fat	Fiber	Sodium	Calories

DAILY TOTALS						
DAILY GOALS						
% DAILY GOALS	%	%	%	%	%	%

WATER   1 cup per circle
(1 cup = 8 ounces ~ 240ml)   ◯ ◯ ◯ ◯ ◯ ◯ ◯ ◯ ◯ ◯ ◯ ◯ ◯ ◯ ◯ ◯

DATE: _____ **WEEK:** _____ **WEIGHT:** _____

BREAKFAST	Protein	Carbs	Fat	Fiber	Sodium	Calories

SNACK	Protein	Carbs	Fat	Fiber	Sodium	Calories

LUNCH	Protein	Carbs	Fat	Fiber	Sodium	Calories

SNACK	Protein	Carbs	Fat	Fiber	Sodium	Calories

DINNER	Protein	Carbs	Fat	Fiber	Sodium	Calories

SNACK	Protein	Carbs	Fat	Fiber	Sodium	Calories

DAILY TOTALS						
DAILY GOALS						
% DAILY GOALS	%	%	%	%	%	%

WATER   1 cup per circle
(1 cup = 8 ounces ~ 240ml)   ◯ ◯ ◯ ◯ ◯ ◯ ◯ ◯ ◯ ◯ ◯ ◯ ◯ ◯ ◯

DATE: [   ]   WEEK: [   ]   WEIGHT: [   ]

BREAKFAST	Protein	Carbs	Fat	Fiber	Sodium	Calories

SNACK	Protein	Carbs	Fat	Fiber	Sodium	Calories

LUNCH	Protein	Carbs	Fat	Fiber	Sodium	Calories

SNACK	Protein	Carbs	Fat	Fiber	Sodium	Calories

DINNER	Protein	Carbs	Fat	Fiber	Sodium	Calories

SNACK	Protein	Carbs	Fat	Fiber	Sodium	Calories

DAILY TOTALS						
DAILY GOALS						
% DAILY GOALS	%	%	%	%	%	%

WATER   1 cup per circle
(1 cup = 8 ounces ~ 240ml)   ○○○○○○○○○○○○○○○○

DATE: _____ **WEEK:** _____ **WEIGHT:** _____

BREAKFAST	Protein	Carbs	Fat	Fiber	Sodium	Calories

SNACK	Protein	Carbs	Fat	Fiber	Sodium	Calories

LUNCH	Protein	Carbs	Fat	Fiber	Sodium	Calories

SNACK	Protein	Carbs	Fat	Fiber	Sodium	Calories

DINNER	Protein	Carbs	Fat	Fiber	Sodium	Calories

SNACK	Protein	Carbs	Fat	Fiber	Sodium	Calories

DAILY TOTALS						
DAILY GOALS						
% DAILY GOALS	%	%	%	%	%	%

WATER   1 cup per circle
(1 cup = 8 ounces ~ 240ml)   ○ ○ ○ ○ ○ ○ ○ ○ ○ ○ ○ ○ ○ ○ ○ ○

DATE: _____ **WEEK:** _____ **WEIGHT:** _____

BREAKFAST	Protein	Carbs	Fat	Fiber	Sodium	Calories

SNACK	Protein	Carbs	Fat	Fiber	Sodium	Calories

LUNCH	Protein	Carbs	Fat	Fiber	Sodium	Calories

SNACK	Protein	Carbs	Fat	Fiber	Sodium	Calories

DINNER	Protein	Carbs	Fat	Fiber	Sodium	Calories

SNACK	Protein	Carbs	Fat	Fiber	Sodium	Calories

DAILY TOTALS						
DAILY GOALS						
% DAILY GOALS	%	%	%	%	%	%

WATER   1 cup per circle
(1 cup = 8 ounces ~ 240ml)   ○○○○○○○○○○○○○○○○○

DATE:	WEEK:	WEIGHT:

BREAKFAST	Protein	Carbs	Fat	Fiber	Sodium	Calories

SNACK	Protein	Carbs	Fat	Fiber	Sodium	Calories

LUNCH	Protein	Carbs	Fat	Fiber	Sodium	Calories

SNACK	Protein	Carbs	Fat	Fiber	Sodium	Calories

DINNER	Protein	Carbs	Fat	Fiber	Sodium	Calories

SNACK	Protein	Carbs	Fat	Fiber	Sodium	Calories

DAILY TOTALS						
DAILY GOALS						
% DAILY GOALS	%	%	%	%	%	%

WATER   1 cup per circle
(1 cup = 8 ounces ~ 240ml)   ○ ○ ○ ○ ○ ○ ○ ○ ○ ○ ○ ○ ○ ○ ○ ○

DATE: [_____] **WEEK:** [_____] **WEIGHT:** [_____]

BREAKFAST	Protein	Carbs	Fat	Fiber	Sodium	Calories

SNACK	Protein	Carbs	Fat	Fiber	Sodium	Calories

LUNCH	Protein	Carbs	Fat	Fiber	Sodium	Calories

SNACK	Protein	Carbs	Fat	Fiber	Sodium	Calories

DINNER	Protein	Carbs	Fat	Fiber	Sodium	Calories

SNACK	Protein	Carbs	Fat	Fiber	Sodium	Calories
DAILY TOTALS						
DAILY GOALS						
% DAILY GOALS	%	%	%	%	%	%

WATER   1 cup per circle
(1 cup = 8 ounces ~ 240ml)   ○○○○○○○○○○○○○○○○

DATE: _____ **WEEK:** _____ **WEIGHT:** _____

BREAKFAST	Protein	Carbs	Fat	Fiber	Sodium	Calories

SNACK	Protein	Carbs	Fat	Fiber	Sodium	Calories

LUNCH	Protein	Carbs	Fat	Fiber	Sodium	Calories

SNACK	Protein	Carbs	Fat	Fiber	Sodium	Calories

DINNER	Protein	Carbs	Fat	Fiber	Sodium	Calories

SNACK	Protein	Carbs	Fat	Fiber	Sodium	Calories

DAILY TOTALS						
DAILY GOALS						
% DAILY GOALS	%	%	%	%	%	%

WATER   1 cup per circle
(1 cup = 8 ounces ~ 240ml)   ○○○○○○○○○○○○○○○○

DATE: _____ **WEEK:** _____ **WEIGHT:** _____

BREAKFAST	Protein	Carbs	Fat	Fiber	Sodium	Calories

SNACK	Protein	Carbs	Fat	Fiber	Sodium	Calories

LUNCH	Protein	Carbs	Fat	Fiber	Sodium	Calories

SNACK	Protein	Carbs	Fat	Fiber	Sodium	Calories

DINNER	Protein	Carbs	Fat	Fiber	Sodium	Calories

SNACK	Protein	Carbs	Fat	Fiber	Sodium	Calories

DAILY TOTALS						
DAILY GOALS						
% DAILY GOALS	%	%	%	%	%	%

WATER   1 cup per circle
(1 cup = 8 ounces ~ 240ml)   ○○○○○○○○○○○○○○○○

DATE:	WEEK:	WEIGHT:

BREAKFAST	Protein	Carbs	Fat	Fiber	Sodium	Calories

SNACK	Protein	Carbs	Fat	Fiber	Sodium	Calories

LUNCH	Protein	Carbs	Fat	Fiber	Sodium	Calories

SNACK	Protein	Carbs	Fat	Fiber	Sodium	Calories

DINNER	Protein	Carbs	Fat	Fiber	Sodium	Calories

SNACK	Protein	Carbs	Fat	Fiber	Sodium	Calories

DAILY TOTALS						
DAILY GOALS						
% DAILY GOALS	%	%	%	%	%	%

WATER   1 cup per circle
(1 cup = 8 ounces ~ 240ml)   ○ ○ ○ ○ ○ ○ ○ ○ ○ ○ ○ ○ ○ ○ ○ ○

DATE:		WEEK:		WEIGHT:	

BREAKFAST	Protein	Carbs	Fat	Fiber	Sodium	Calories

SNACK	Protein	Carbs	Fat	Fiber	Sodium	Calories

LUNCH	Protein	Carbs	Fat	Fiber	Sodium	Calories

SNACK	Protein	Carbs	Fat	Fiber	Sodium	Calories

DINNER	Protein	Carbs	Fat	Fiber	Sodium	Calories

SNACK	Protein	Carbs	Fat	Fiber	Sodium	Calories
DAILY TOTALS						
DAILY GOALS						
% DAILY GOALS	%	%	%	%	%	%

WATER   1 cup per circle
(1 cup = 8 ounces ~ 240ml)   ○ ○ ○ ○ ○ ○ ○ ○ ○ ○ ○ ○ ○ ○ ○ ○

DATE: _____ **WEEK:** _____ **WEIGHT:** _____

BREAKFAST	Protein	Carbs	Fat	Fiber	Sodium	Calories

SNACK	Protein	Carbs	Fat	Fiber	Sodium	Calories

LUNCH	Protein	Carbs	Fat	Fiber	Sodium	Calories

SNACK	Protein	Carbs	Fat	Fiber	Sodium	Calories

DINNER	Protein	Carbs	Fat	Fiber	Sodium	Calories

SNACK	Protein	Carbs	Fat	Fiber	Sodium	Calories

DAILY TOTALS						
DAILY GOALS						
% DAILY GOALS	%	%	%	%	%	%

WATER 1 cup per circle
(1 cup = 8 ounces ~ 240ml)   ◯ ◯ ◯ ◯ ◯ ◯ ◯ ◯ ◯ ◯ ◯ ◯ ◯ ◯ ◯ ◯

DATE:		WEEK:		WEIGHT:	

BREAKFAST	Protein	Carbs	Fat	Fiber	Sodium	Calories

SNACK	Protein	Carbs	Fat	Fiber	Sodium	Calories

LUNCH	Protein	Carbs	Fat	Fiber	Sodium	Calories

SNACK	Protein	Carbs	Fat	Fiber	Sodium	Calories

DINNER	Protein	Carbs	Fat	Fiber	Sodium	Calories

SNACK	Protein	Carbs	Fat	Fiber	Sodium	Calories

DAILY TOTALS						
DAILY GOALS						
% DAILY GOALS	%	%	%	%	%	%

WATER   1 cup per circle
(1 cup = 8 ounces ~ 240ml)   ○○○○○○○○○○○○○○○○

DATE: _____ **WEEK:** _____ **WEIGHT:** _____

BREAKFAST	Protein	Carbs	Fat	Fiber	Sodium	Calories

SNACK	Protein	Carbs	Fat	Fiber	Sodium	Calories

LUNCH	Protein	Carbs	Fat	Fiber	Sodium	Calories

SNACK	Protein	Carbs	Fat	Fiber	Sodium	Calories

DINNER	Protein	Carbs	Fat	Fiber	Sodium	Calories

SNACK	Protein	Carbs	Fat	Fiber	Sodium	Calories

DAILY TOTALS						
DAILY GOALS						
% DAILY GOALS	%	%	%	%	%	%

WATER   1 cup per circle
(1 cup = 8 ounces ~ 240ml)   ○ ○ ○ ○ ○ ○ ○ ○ ○ ○ ○ ○ ○ ○

DATE: _____ **WEEK:** _____ **WEIGHT:** _____

BREAKFAST	Protein	Carbs	Fat	Fiber	Sodium	Calories

SNACK	Protein	Carbs	Fat	Fiber	Sodium	Calories

LUNCH	Protein	Carbs	Fat	Fiber	Sodium	Calories

SNACK	Protein	Carbs	Fat	Fiber	Sodium	Calories

DINNER	Protein	Carbs	Fat	Fiber	Sodium	Calories

SNACK	Protein	Carbs	Fat	Fiber	Sodium	Calories

DAILY TOTALS						
DAILY GOALS						
% DAILY GOALS	%	%	%	%	%	%

WATER   1 cup per circle
(1 cup = 8 ounces ~ 240ml)   ○ ○ ○ ○ ○ ○ ○ ○ ○ ○ ○ ○ ○ ○ ○

DATE: _____ **WEEK:** _____ **WEIGHT:** _____

BREAKFAST	Protein	Carbs	Fat	Fiber	Sodium	Calories

SNACK	Protein	Carbs	Fat	Fiber	Sodium	Calories

LUNCH	Protein	Carbs	Fat	Fiber	Sodium	Calories

SNACK	Protein	Carbs	Fat	Fiber	Sodium	Calories

DINNER	Protein	Carbs	Fat	Fiber	Sodium	Calories

SNACK	Protein	Carbs	Fat	Fiber	Sodium	Calories

DAILY TOTALS						
DAILY GOALS						
% DAILY GOALS	%	%	%	%	%	%

WATER   1 cup per circle
(1 cup = 8 ounces ~ 240ml)   ◯◯◯◯◯◯◯◯◯◯◯◯◯◯◯◯

DATE: _____ **WEEK:** _____ **WEIGHT:** _____

BREAKFAST	Protein	Carbs	Fat	Fiber	Sodium	Calories

SNACK	Protein	Carbs	Fat	Fiber	Sodium	Calories

LUNCH	Protein	Carbs	Fat	Fiber	Sodium	Calories

SNACK	Protein	Carbs	Fat	Fiber	Sodium	Calories

DINNER	Protein	Carbs	Fat	Fiber	Sodium	Calories

SNACK	Protein	Carbs	Fat	Fiber	Sodium	Calories

	Protein	Carbs	Fat	Fiber	Sodium	Calories
DAILY TOTALS						
DAILY GOALS						
% DAILY GOALS	%	%	%	%	%	%

WATER   1 cup per circle
(1 cup = 8 ounces ~ 240ml)   ○ ○ ○ ○ ○ ○ ○ ○ ○ ○ ○ ○ ○ ○ ○

DATE:	WEEK:	WEIGHT:

BREAKFAST	Protein	Carbs	Fat	Fiber	Sodium	Calories

SNACK	Protein	Carbs	Fat	Fiber	Sodium	Calories

LUNCH	Protein	Carbs	Fat	Fiber	Sodium	Calories

SNACK	Protein	Carbs	Fat	Fiber	Sodium	Calories

DINNER	Protein	Carbs	Fat	Fiber	Sodium	Calories

SNACK	Protein	Carbs	Fat	Fiber	Sodium	Calories

	Protein	Carbs	Fat	Fiber	Sodium	Calories
DAILY TOTALS						
DAILY GOALS						
% DAILY GOALS	%	%	%	%	%	%

WATER   1 cup per circle
(1 cup = 8 ounces ~ 240ml)   ○ ○ ○ ○ ○ ○ ○ ○ ○ ○ ○ ○ ○ ○ ○ ○

DATE: _____ **WEEK:** _____ **WEIGHT:** _____

BREAKFAST	Protein	Carbs	Fat	Fiber	Sodium	Calories

SNACK	Protein	Carbs	Fat	Fiber	Sodium	Calories

LUNCH	Protein	Carbs	Fat	Fiber	Sodium	Calories

SNACK	Protein	Carbs	Fat	Fiber	Sodium	Calories

DINNER	Protein	Carbs	Fat	Fiber	Sodium	Calories

SNACK	Protein	Carbs	Fat	Fiber	Sodium	Calories

DAILY TOTALS						
DAILY GOALS						
% DAILY GOALS	%	%	%	%	%	%

WATER   1 cup per circle
(1 cup = 8 ounces ~ 240ml)   ○ ○ ○ ○ ○ ○ ○ ○ ○ ○ ○ ○ ○ ○ ○

DATE: _____ **WEEK:** _____ **WEIGHT:** _____

BREAKFAST	Protein	Carbs	Fat	Fiber	Sodium	Calories

SNACK	Protein	Carbs	Fat	Fiber	Sodium	Calories

LUNCH	Protein	Carbs	Fat	Fiber	Sodium	Calories

SNACK	Protein	Carbs	Fat	Fiber	Sodium	Calories

DINNER	Protein	Carbs	Fat	Fiber	Sodium	Calories

SNACK	Protein	Carbs	Fat	Fiber	Sodium	Calories

DAILY TOTALS						
DAILY GOALS						
% DAILY GOALS	%	%	%	%	%	%

WATER   1 cup per circle
(1 cup = 8 ounces ~ 240ml)   ○ ○ ○ ○ ○ ○ ○ ○ ○ ○ ○ ○ ○ ○ ○ ○

DATE: _____ **WEEK:** _____ **WEIGHT:** _____

BREAKFAST	Protein	Carbs	Fat	Fiber	Sodium	Calories

SNACK	Protein	Carbs	Fat	Fiber	Sodium	Calories

LUNCH	Protein	Carbs	Fat	Fiber	Sodium	Calories

SNACK	Protein	Carbs	Fat	Fiber	Sodium	Calories

DINNER	Protein	Carbs	Fat	Fiber	Sodium	Calories

SNACK	Protein	Carbs	Fat	Fiber	Sodium	Calories

DAILY TOTALS						
DAILY GOALS						
% DAILY GOALS	%	%	%	%	%	%

WATER   1 cup per circle
(1 cup = 8 ounces ~ 240ml)   ◯ ◯ ◯ ◯ ◯ ◯ ◯ ◯ ◯ ◯ ◯ ◯ ◯ ◯

DATE: | **WEEK:** | **WEIGHT:**

BREAKFAST	Protein	Carbs	Fat	Fiber	Sodium	Calories

SNACK	Protein	Carbs	Fat	Fiber	Sodium	Calories

LUNCH	Protein	Carbs	Fat	Fiber	Sodium	Calories

SNACK	Protein	Carbs	Fat	Fiber	Sodium	Calories

DINNER	Protein	Carbs	Fat	Fiber	Sodium	Calories

SNACK	Protein	Carbs	Fat	Fiber	Sodium	Calories

DAILY TOTALS						
DAILY GOALS						
% DAILY GOALS	%	%	%	%	%	%

WATER   1 cup per circle
(1 cup = 8 ounces ~ 240ml)   ◯ ◯ ◯ ◯ ◯ ◯ ◯ ◯ ◯ ◯ ◯ ◯ ◯ ◯ ◯

DATE: [   ]   **WEEK:** [   ]   **WEIGHT:** [   ]

BREAKFAST	Protein	Carbs	Fat	Fiber	Sodium	Calories

SNACK	Protein	Carbs	Fat	Fiber	Sodium	Calories

LUNCH	Protein	Carbs	Fat	Fiber	Sodium	Calories

SNACK	Protein	Carbs	Fat	Fiber	Sodium	Calories

DINNER	Protein	Carbs	Fat	Fiber	Sodium	Calories

SNACK	Protein	Carbs	Fat	Fiber	Sodium	Calories

DAILY TOTALS						
DAILY GOALS						
% DAILY GOALS	%	%	%	%	%	%

WATER   1 cup per circle
(1 cup = 8 ounces ~ 240ml)   ○○○○○○○○○○○○○○○

DATE: _____ **WEEK:** _____ **WEIGHT:** _____

BREAKFAST	Protein	Carbs	Fat	Fiber	Sodium	Calories

SNACK	Protein	Carbs	Fat	Fiber	Sodium	Calories

LUNCH	Protein	Carbs	Fat	Fiber	Sodium	Calories

SNACK	Protein	Carbs	Fat	Fiber	Sodium	Calories

DINNER	Protein	Carbs	Fat	Fiber	Sodium	Calories

SNACK	Protein	Carbs	Fat	Fiber	Sodium	Calories

DAILY TOTALS						
DAILY GOALS						
% DAILY GOALS	%	%	%	%	%	%

WATER   1 cup per circle
(1 cup = 8 ounces ~ 240ml)   ○○○○○○○○○○○○○○○○○○

DATE: _____   **WEEK:** _____   **WEIGHT:** _____

BREAKFAST	Protein	Carbs	Fat	Fiber	Sodium	Calories

SNACK	Protein	Carbs	Fat	Fiber	Sodium	Calories

LUNCH	Protein	Carbs	Fat	Fiber	Sodium	Calories

SNACK	Protein	Carbs	Fat	Fiber	Sodium	Calories

DINNER	Protein	Carbs	Fat	Fiber	Sodium	Calories

SNACK	Protein	Carbs	Fat	Fiber	Sodium	Calories

DAILY TOTALS						
DAILY GOALS						
% DAILY GOALS	%	%	%	%	%	%

WATER   1 cup per circle
(1 cup = 8 ounces ~ 240ml)   ○○○○○○○○○○○○○○○○

DATE: _____ **WEEK:** _____ **WEIGHT:** _____

BREAKFAST	Protein	Carbs	Fat	Fiber	Sodium	Calories
SNACK	**Protein**	**Carbs**	**Fat**	**Fiber**	**Sodium**	**Calories**
LUNCH	**Protein**	**Carbs**	**Fat**	**Fiber**	**Sodium**	**Calories**
SNACK	**Protein**	**Carbs**	**Fat**	**Fiber**	**Sodium**	**Calories**
DINNER	**Protein**	**Carbs**	**Fat**	**Fiber**	**Sodium**	**Calories**
SNACK	**Protein**	**Carbs**	**Fat**	**Fiber**	**Sodium**	**Calories**
DAILY TOTALS						
DAILY GOALS						
% DAILY GOALS	%	%	%	%	%	%

WATER   1 cup per circle
(1 cup = 8 ounces ~ 240ml)   ○ ○ ○ ○ ○ ○ ○ ○ ○ ○ ○ ○ ○ ○

DATE:	WEEK:	WEIGHT:

BREAKFAST	Protein	Carbs	Fat	Fiber	Sodium	Calories

SNACK	Protein	Carbs	Fat	Fiber	Sodium	Calories

LUNCH	Protein	Carbs	Fat	Fiber	Sodium	Calories

SNACK	Protein	Carbs	Fat	Fiber	Sodium	Calories

DINNER	Protein	Carbs	Fat	Fiber	Sodium	Calories

SNACK	Protein	Carbs	Fat	Fiber	Sodium	Calories

DAILY TOTALS						
DAILY GOALS						
% DAILY GOALS	%	%	%	%	%	%

**WATER   1 cup per circle
(1 cup = 8 ounces ~ 240ml)**   ◯ ◯ ◯ ◯ ◯ ◯ ◯ ◯ ◯ ◯ ◯ ◯ ◯ ◯ ◯

DATE: _____ **WEEK:** _____ **WEIGHT:** _____

BREAKFAST	Protein	Carbs	Fat	Fiber	Sodium	Calories

SNACK	Protein	Carbs	Fat	Fiber	Sodium	Calories

LUNCH	Protein	Carbs	Fat	Fiber	Sodium	Calories

SNACK	Protein	Carbs	Fat	Fiber	Sodium	Calories

DINNER	Protein	Carbs	Fat	Fiber	Sodium	Calories

SNACK	Protein	Carbs	Fat	Fiber	Sodium	Calories

DAILY TOTALS						
DAILY GOALS						
% DAILY GOALS	%	%	%	%	%	%

WATER   1 cup per circle
(1 cup = 8 ounces ~ 240ml)   ○ ○ ○ ○ ○ ○ ○ ○ ○ ○ ○ ○ ○ ○ ○ ○ ○ ○

DATE: [   ]   **WEEK:** [   ]   **WEIGHT:** [   ]

BREAKFAST	Protein	Carbs	Fat	Fiber	Sodium	Calories

SNACK	Protein	Carbs	Fat	Fiber	Sodium	Calories

LUNCH	Protein	Carbs	Fat	Fiber	Sodium	Calories

SNACK	Protein	Carbs	Fat	Fiber	Sodium	Calories

DINNER	Protein	Carbs	Fat	Fiber	Sodium	Calories

SNACK	Protein	Carbs	Fat	Fiber	Sodium	Calories

DAILY TOTALS						
DAILY GOALS						
% DAILY GOALS	%	%	%	%	%	%

WATER   1 cup per circle
(1 cup = 8 ounces ~ 240ml)   ◯◯◯◯◯◯◯◯◯◯◯◯◯◯◯◯

DATE: [_____]   **WEEK:** [_____]   **WEIGHT:** [_____]

BREAKFAST	Protein	Carbs	Fat	Fiber	Sodium	Calories

SNACK	Protein	Carbs	Fat	Fiber	Sodium	Calories

LUNCH	Protein	Carbs	Fat	Fiber	Sodium	Calories

SNACK	Protein	Carbs	Fat	Fiber	Sodium	Calories

DINNER	Protein	Carbs	Fat	Fiber	Sodium	Calories

SNACK	Protein	Carbs	Fat	Fiber	Sodium	Calories

DAILY TOTALS						
DAILY GOALS						
% DAILY GOALS	%	%	%	%	%	%

WATER   1 cup per circle
(1 cup = 8 ounces ~ 240ml)   ○ ○ ○ ○ ○ ○ ○ ○ ○ ○ ○ ○ ○ ○ ○ ○

DATE:	WEEK:	WEIGHT:

BREAKFAST	Protein	Carbs	Fat	Fiber	Sodium	Calories

SNACK	Protein	Carbs	Fat	Fiber	Sodium	Calories

LUNCH	Protein	Carbs	Fat	Fiber	Sodium	Calories

SNACK	Protein	Carbs	Fat	Fiber	Sodium	Calories

DINNER	Protein	Carbs	Fat	Fiber	Sodium	Calories

SNACK	Protein	Carbs	Fat	Fiber	Sodium	Calories

DAILY TOTALS						
DAILY GOALS						
% DAILY GOALS	%	%	%	%	%	%

**WATER   1 cup per circle
(1 cup = 8 ounces ~ 240ml)**   ○ ○ ○ ○ ○ ○ ○ ○ ○ ○ ○ ○ ○ ○ ○

DATE: _____ **WEEK:** _____ **WEIGHT:** _____

BREAKFAST	Protein	Carbs	Fat	Fiber	Sodium	Calories

SNACK	Protein	Carbs	Fat	Fiber	Sodium	Calories

LUNCH	Protein	Carbs	Fat	Fiber	Sodium	Calories

SNACK	Protein	Carbs	Fat	Fiber	Sodium	Calories

DINNER	Protein	Carbs	Fat	Fiber	Sodium	Calories

SNACK	Protein	Carbs	Fat	Fiber	Sodium	Calories

DAILY TOTALS						
DAILY GOALS						
% DAILY GOALS	%	%	%	%	%	%

WATER 1 cup per circle
(1 cup = 8 ounces ~ 240ml)   ○ ○ ○ ○ ○ ○ ○ ○ ○ ○ ○ ○ ○ ○ ○ ○

DATE: _____   **WEEK:** _____   **WEIGHT:** _____

BREAKFAST	Protein	Carbs	Fat	Fiber	Sodium	Calories

SNACK	Protein	Carbs	Fat	Fiber	Sodium	Calories

LUNCH	Protein	Carbs	Fat	Fiber	Sodium	Calories

SNACK	Protein	Carbs	Fat	Fiber	Sodium	Calories

DINNER	Protein	Carbs	Fat	Fiber	Sodium	Calories

SNACK	Protein	Carbs	Fat	Fiber	Sodium	Calories

DAILY TOTALS						
DAILY GOALS						
% DAILY GOALS	%	%	%	%	%	%

WATER 1 cup per circle
(1 cup = 8 ounces ~ 240ml) ○○○○○○○○○○○○○○○○

DATE: _____ WEEK: _____ WEIGHT: _____

BREAKFAST	Protein	Carbs	Fat	Fiber	Sodium	Calories

SNACK	Protein	Carbs	Fat	Fiber	Sodium	Calories

LUNCH	Protein	Carbs	Fat	Fiber	Sodium	Calories

SNACK	Protein	Carbs	Fat	Fiber	Sodium	Calories

DINNER	Protein	Carbs	Fat	Fiber	Sodium	Calories

SNACK	Protein	Carbs	Fat	Fiber	Sodium	Calories

DAILY TOTALS						
DAILY GOALS						
% DAILY GOALS	%	%	%	%	%	%

WATER 1 cup per circle
(1 cup = 8 ounces ~ 240ml)   ○○○○○○○○○○○○○○○○○○

DATE: _____ WEEK: _____ WEIGHT: _____

BREAKFAST	Protein	Carbs	Fat	Fiber	Sodium	Calories

SNACK	Protein	Carbs	Fat	Fiber	Sodium	Calories

LUNCH	Protein	Carbs	Fat	Fiber	Sodium	Calories

SNACK	Protein	Carbs	Fat	Fiber	Sodium	Calories

DINNER	Protein	Carbs	Fat	Fiber	Sodium	Calories

SNACK	Protein	Carbs	Fat	Fiber	Sodium	Calories
DAILY TOTALS						
DAILY GOALS						
% DAILY GOALS	%	%	%	%	%	%

WATER   1 cup per circle
(1 cup = 8 ounces ~ 240ml)   ○○○○○○○○○○○○○○○○

DATE: _____ WEEK: _____ WEIGHT: _____

BREAKFAST	Protein	Carbs	Fat	Fiber	Sodium	Calories

SNACK	Protein	Carbs	Fat	Fiber	Sodium	Calories

LUNCH	Protein	Carbs	Fat	Fiber	Sodium	Calories

SNACK	Protein	Carbs	Fat	Fiber	Sodium	Calories

DINNER	Protein	Carbs	Fat	Fiber	Sodium	Calories

SNACK	Protein	Carbs	Fat	Fiber	Sodium	Calories

DAILY TOTALS						
DAILY GOALS						
% DAILY GOALS	%	%	%	%	%	%

WATER 1 cup per circle
(1 cup = 8 ounces ~ 240ml)   ○ ○ ○ ○ ○ ○ ○ ○ ○ ○ ○ ○ ○ ○ ○ ○

DATE: _____ **WEEK:** _____ **WEIGHT:** _____

BREAKFAST	Protein	Carbs	Fat	Fiber	Sodium	Calories

SNACK	Protein	Carbs	Fat	Fiber	Sodium	Calories

LUNCH	Protein	Carbs	Fat	Fiber	Sodium	Calories

SNACK	Protein	Carbs	Fat	Fiber	Sodium	Calories

DINNER	Protein	Carbs	Fat	Fiber	Sodium	Calories

SNACK	Protein	Carbs	Fat	Fiber	Sodium	Calories

DAILY TOTALS						
DAILY GOALS						
% DAILY GOALS	%	%	%	%	%	%

WATER   1 cup per circle
(1 cup = 8 ounces ~ 240ml)   ○○○○○○○○○○○○○○○○

DATE:		WEEK:		WEIGHT:			

BREAKFAST	Protein	Carbs	Fat	Fiber	Sodium	Calories

SNACK	Protein	Carbs	Fat	Fiber	Sodium	Calories

LUNCH	Protein	Carbs	Fat	Fiber	Sodium	Calories

SNACK	Protein	Carbs	Fat	Fiber	Sodium	Calories

DINNER	Protein	Carbs	Fat	Fiber	Sodium	Calories

SNACK	Protein	Carbs	Fat	Fiber	Sodium	Calories

DAILY TOTALS						
DAILY GOALS						
% DAILY GOALS	%	%	%	%	%	%

WATER   1 cup per circle
(1 cup = 8 ounces ~ 240ml)   ○○○○○○○○○○○○○○○○○○○

DATE: [   ]   **WEEK:** [   ]   **WEIGHT:** [   ]

BREAKFAST	Protein	Carbs	Fat	Fiber	Sodium	Calories

SNACK	Protein	Carbs	Fat	Fiber	Sodium	Calories

LUNCH	Protein	Carbs	Fat	Fiber	Sodium	Calories

SNACK	Protein	Carbs	Fat	Fiber	Sodium	Calories

DINNER	Protein	Carbs	Fat	Fiber	Sodium	Calories

SNACK	Protein	Carbs	Fat	Fiber	Sodium	Calories

DAILY TOTALS						
DAILY GOALS						
% DAILY GOALS	%	%	%	%	%	%

WATER   1 cup per circle
(1 cup = 8 ounces ~ 240ml)   ◯◯◯◯◯◯◯◯◯◯◯◯◯◯◯◯

DATE: _____ **WEEK:** _____ **WEIGHT:** _____

BREAKFAST	Protein	Carbs	Fat	Fiber	Sodium	Calories

SNACK	Protein	Carbs	Fat	Fiber	Sodium	Calories

LUNCH	Protein	Carbs	Fat	Fiber	Sodium	Calories

SNACK	Protein	Carbs	Fat	Fiber	Sodium	Calories

DINNER	Protein	Carbs	Fat	Fiber	Sodium	Calories

SNACK	Protein	Carbs	Fat	Fiber	Sodium	Calories

DAILY TOTALS						
DAILY GOALS						
% DAILY GOALS	%	%	%	%	%	%

WATER   1 cup per circle
(1 cup = 8 ounces ~ 240ml)   ○○○○○○○○○○○○○○○○

DATE: _____   **WEEK:** _____   **WEIGHT:** _____

BREAKFAST	Protein	Carbs	Fat	Fiber	Sodium	Calories

SNACK	Protein	Carbs	Fat	Fiber	Sodium	Calories

LUNCH	Protein	Carbs	Fat	Fiber	Sodium	Calories

SNACK	Protein	Carbs	Fat	Fiber	Sodium	Calories

DINNER	Protein	Carbs	Fat	Fiber	Sodium	Calories

SNACK	Protein	Carbs	Fat	Fiber	Sodium	Calories

DAILY TOTALS						
DAILY GOALS						
% DAILY GOALS	%	%	%	%	%	%

WATER 1 cup per circle
(1 cup = 8 ounces ~ 240ml)   ○○○○○○○○○○○○○○○○

DATE:		WEEK:		WEIGHT:			

BREAKFAST	Protein	Carbs	Fat	Fiber	Sodium	Calories

SNACK	Protein	Carbs	Fat	Fiber	Sodium	Calories

LUNCH	Protein	Carbs	Fat	Fiber	Sodium	Calories

SNACK	Protein	Carbs	Fat	Fiber	Sodium	Calories

DINNER	Protein	Carbs	Fat	Fiber	Sodium	Calories

SNACK	Protein	Carbs	Fat	Fiber	Sodium	Calories

DAILY TOTALS						
DAILY GOALS						
% DAILY GOALS	%	%	%	%	%	%

WATER   1 cup per circle
(1 cup = 8 ounces ~ 240ml)   ○○○○○○○○○○○○○○○

DATE: _____ **WEEK:** _____ **WEIGHT:** _____

BREAKFAST	Protein	Carbs	Fat	Fiber	Sodium	Calories

SNACK	Protein	Carbs	Fat	Fiber	Sodium	Calories

LUNCH	Protein	Carbs	Fat	Fiber	Sodium	Calories

SNACK	Protein	Carbs	Fat	Fiber	Sodium	Calories

DINNER	Protein	Carbs	Fat	Fiber	Sodium	Calories

SNACK	Protein	Carbs	Fat	Fiber	Sodium	Calories

	Protein	Carbs	Fat	Fiber	Sodium	Calories
DAILY TOTALS						
DAILY GOALS						
% DAILY GOALS	%	%	%	%	%	%

WATER 1 cup per circle
(1 cup = 8 ounces ~ 240ml) ○ ○ ○ ○ ○ ○ ○ ○ ○ ○ ○ ○ ○ ○ ○ ○

DATE: _____ **WEEK:** _____ **WEIGHT:** _____

BREAKFAST	Protein	Carbs	Fat	Fiber	Sodium	Calories

SNACK	Protein	Carbs	Fat	Fiber	Sodium	Calories

LUNCH	Protein	Carbs	Fat	Fiber	Sodium	Calories

SNACK	Protein	Carbs	Fat	Fiber	Sodium	Calories

DINNER	Protein	Carbs	Fat	Fiber	Sodium	Calories

SNACK	Protein	Carbs	Fat	Fiber	Sodium	Calories

	Protein	Carbs	Fat	Fiber	Sodium	Calories
DAILY TOTALS						
DAILY GOALS						
% DAILY GOALS	%	%	%	%	%	%

WATER   1 cup per circle
(1 cup = 8 ounces ~ 240ml)   ○○○○○○○○○○○○○○○○○○

DATE: **WEEK:** **WEIGHT:**

BREAKFAST	Protein	Carbs	Fat	Fiber	Sodium	Calories

SNACK	Protein	Carbs	Fat	Fiber	Sodium	Calories

LUNCH	Protein	Carbs	Fat	Fiber	Sodium	Calories

SNACK	Protein	Carbs	Fat	Fiber	Sodium	Calories

DINNER	Protein	Carbs	Fat	Fiber	Sodium	Calories

SNACK	Protein	Carbs	Fat	Fiber	Sodium	Calories
DAILY TOTALS						
DAILY GOALS						
% DAILY GOALS	%	%	%	%	%	%

WATER 1 cup per circle
(1 cup = 8 ounces ~ 240ml)   ○○○○○○○○○○○○○○○○○

DATE: _____   **WEEK:** _____   **WEIGHT:** _____

BREAKFAST	Protein	Carbs	Fat	Fiber	Sodium	Calories

SNACK	Protein	Carbs	Fat	Fiber	Sodium	Calories

LUNCH	Protein	Carbs	Fat	Fiber	Sodium	Calories

SNACK	Protein	Carbs	Fat	Fiber	Sodium	Calories

DINNER	Protein	Carbs	Fat	Fiber	Sodium	Calories

SNACK	Protein	Carbs	Fat	Fiber	Sodium	Calories
DAILY TOTALS						
DAILY GOALS						
% DAILY GOALS	%	%	%	%	%	%

WATER   1 cup per circle
(1 cup = 8 ounces ~ 240ml)   ○○○○○○○○○○○○○○○○○○

DATE: _____ **WEEK:** _____ **WEIGHT:** _____

BREAKFAST	Protein	Carbs	Fat	Fiber	Sodium	Calories

SNACK	Protein	Carbs	Fat	Fiber	Sodium	Calories

LUNCH	Protein	Carbs	Fat	Fiber	Sodium	Calories

SNACK	Protein	Carbs	Fat	Fiber	Sodium	Calories

DINNER	Protein	Carbs	Fat	Fiber	Sodium	Calories

SNACK	Protein	Carbs	Fat	Fiber	Sodium	Calories

DAILY TOTALS						
DAILY GOALS						
% DAILY GOALS	%	%	%	%	%	%

WATER   1 cup per circle
(1 cup = 8 ounces ~ 240ml)   ○ ○ ○ ○ ○ ○ ○ ○ ○ ○ ○ ○ ○ ○ ○ ○

DATE: [ ]   WEEK: [ ]   WEIGHT: [ ]

BREAKFAST	Protein	Carbs	Fat	Fiber	Sodium	Calories

SNACK	Protein	Carbs	Fat	Fiber	Sodium	Calories

LUNCH	Protein	Carbs	Fat	Fiber	Sodium	Calories

SNACK	Protein	Carbs	Fat	Fiber	Sodium	Calories

DINNER	Protein	Carbs	Fat	Fiber	Sodium	Calories

SNACK	Protein	Carbs	Fat	Fiber	Sodium	Calories

DAILY TOTALS						
DAILY GOALS						
% DAILY GOALS	%	%	%	%	%	%

WATER   1 cup per circle
(1 cup = 8 ounces ~ 240ml)   ○○○○○○○○○○○○○○○○○○○

DATE: WEEK: WEIGHT:

BREAKFAST	Protein	Carbs	Fat	Fiber	Sodium	Calories

SNACK	Protein	Carbs	Fat	Fiber	Sodium	Calories

LUNCH	Protein	Carbs	Fat	Fiber	Sodium	Calories

SNACK	Protein	Carbs	Fat	Fiber	Sodium	Calories

DINNER	Protein	Carbs	Fat	Fiber	Sodium	Calories

SNACK	Protein	Carbs	Fat	Fiber	Sodium	Calories

DAILY TOTALS						
DAILY GOALS						
% DAILY GOALS	%	%	%	%	%	%

WATER   1 cup per circle
(1 cup = 8 ounces ~ 240ml)   ○○○○○○○○○○○○○○○○

DATE: [   ]   **WEEK:** [   ]   **WEIGHT:** [   ]

BREAKFAST	Protein	Carbs	Fat	Fiber	Sodium	Calories

SNACK	Protein	Carbs	Fat	Fiber	Sodium	Calories

LUNCH	Protein	Carbs	Fat	Fiber	Sodium	Calories

SNACK	Protein	Carbs	Fat	Fiber	Sodium	Calories

DINNER	Protein	Carbs	Fat	Fiber	Sodium	Calories

SNACK	Protein	Carbs	Fat	Fiber	Sodium	Calories

DAILY TOTALS						
DAILY GOALS						
% DAILY GOALS	%	%	%	%	%	%

WATER   1 cup per circle
(1 cup = 8 ounces ~ 240ml)   ○○○○○○○○○○○○○○○○

DATE: [　　　　]　　**WEEK:** [　]　　**WEIGHT:** [　　　　]

BREAKFAST	Protein	Carbs	Fat	Fiber	Sodium	Calories

SNACK	Protein	Carbs	Fat	Fiber	Sodium	Calories

LUNCH	Protein	Carbs	Fat	Fiber	Sodium	Calories

SNACK	Protein	Carbs	Fat	Fiber	Sodium	Calories

DINNER	Protein	Carbs	Fat	Fiber	Sodium	Calories

SNACK	Protein	Carbs	Fat	Fiber	Sodium	Calories

DAILY TOTALS						
DAILY GOALS						
% DAILY GOALS	%	%	%	%	%	%

WATER　1 cup per circle
(1 cup = 8 ounces ~ 240ml)　○○○○○○○○○○○○○○○○○○

DATE: **WEEK:**   **WEIGHT:**

BREAKFAST	Protein	Carbs	Fat	Fiber	Sodium	Calories

SNACK	Protein	Carbs	Fat	Fiber	Sodium	Calories

LUNCH	Protein	Carbs	Fat	Fiber	Sodium	Calories

SNACK	Protein	Carbs	Fat	Fiber	Sodium	Calories

DINNER	Protein	Carbs	Fat	Fiber	Sodium	Calories

SNACK	Protein	Carbs	Fat	Fiber	Sodium	Calories
DAILY TOTALS						
DAILY GOALS						
% DAILY GOALS	%	%	%	%	%	%

WATER   1 cup per circle
(1 cup = 8 ounces ~ 240ml)

○ ○ ○ ○ ○ ○ ○ ○ ○ ○ ○ ○ ○ ○ ○ ○

DATE:	WEEK:	WEIGHT:

BREAKFAST	Protein	Carbs	Fat	Fiber	Sodium	Calories

SNACK	Protein	Carbs	Fat	Fiber	Sodium	Calories

LUNCH	Protein	Carbs	Fat	Fiber	Sodium	Calories

SNACK	Protein	Carbs	Fat	Fiber	Sodium	Calories

DINNER	Protein	Carbs	Fat	Fiber	Sodium	Calories

SNACK	Protein	Carbs	Fat	Fiber	Sodium	Calories

DAILY TOTALS						
DAILY GOALS						
% DAILY GOALS	%	%	%	%	%	%

WATER 1 cup per circle
(1 cup = 8 ounces ~ 240ml)   ○○○○○○○○○○○○○○○○

DATE: [   ]   WEEK: [   ]   WEIGHT: [   ]

BREAKFAST	Protein	Carbs	Fat	Fiber	Sodium	Calories

SNACK	Protein	Carbs	Fat	Fiber	Sodium	Calories

LUNCH	Protein	Carbs	Fat	Fiber	Sodium	Calories

SNACK	Protein	Carbs	Fat	Fiber	Sodium	Calories

DINNER	Protein	Carbs	Fat	Fiber	Sodium	Calories

SNACK	Protein	Carbs	Fat	Fiber	Sodium	Calories
DAILY TOTALS						
DAILY GOALS						
% DAILY GOALS	%	%	%	%	%	%

WATER   1 cup per circle
(1 cup = 8 ounces ~ 240ml)   ○○○○○○○○○○○○○○○○○○

DATE:	WEEK:	WEIGHT:

BREAKFAST	Protein	Carbs	Fat	Fiber	Sodium	Calories
SNACK	Protein	Carbs	Fat	Fiber	Sodium	Calories
LUNCH	Protein	Carbs	Fat	Fiber	Sodium	Calories
SNACK	Protein	Carbs	Fat	Fiber	Sodium	Calories
DINNER	Protein	Carbs	Fat	Fiber	Sodium	Calories
SNACK	Protein	Carbs	Fat	Fiber	Sodium	Calories
DAILY TOTALS						
DAILY GOALS						
% DAILY GOALS	%	%	%	%	%	%

WATER   1 cup per circle
(1 cup = 8 ounces ~ 240ml)   ○ ○ ○ ○ ○ ○ ○ ○ ○ ○ ○ ○ ○ ○ ○

DATE: [   ]   **WEEK:** [   ]   **WEIGHT:** [   ]

BREAKFAST	Protein	Carbs	Fat	Fiber	Sodium	Calories

SNACK	Protein	Carbs	Fat	Fiber	Sodium	Calories

LUNCH	Protein	Carbs	Fat	Fiber	Sodium	Calories

SNACK	Protein	Carbs	Fat	Fiber	Sodium	Calories

DINNER	Protein	Carbs	Fat	Fiber	Sodium	Calories

SNACK	Protein	Carbs	Fat	Fiber	Sodium	Calories
DAILY TOTALS						
DAILY GOALS						
% DAILY GOALS	%	%	%	%	%	%

WATER   1 cup per circle
(1 cup = 8 ounces ~ 240ml)   ○○○○○○○○○○○○○○○○

DATE: _____ **WEEK:** _____ **WEIGHT:** _____

BREAKFAST	Protein	Carbs	Fat	Fiber	Sodium	Calories

SNACK	Protein	Carbs	Fat	Fiber	Sodium	Calories

LUNCH	Protein	Carbs	Fat	Fiber	Sodium	Calories

SNACK	Protein	Carbs	Fat	Fiber	Sodium	Calories

DINNER	Protein	Carbs	Fat	Fiber	Sodium	Calories

SNACK	Protein	Carbs	Fat	Fiber	Sodium	Calories

DAILY TOTALS						
DAILY GOALS						
% DAILY GOALS	%	%	%	%	%	%

WATER   1 cup per circle
(1 cup = 8 ounces ~ 240ml)

○ ○ ○ ○ ○ ○ ○ ○ ○ ○ ○ ○ ○ ○ ○ ○

DATE: _____ WEEK: _____ WEIGHT: _____

BREAKFAST	Protein	Carbs	Fat	Fiber	Sodium	Calories

SNACK	Protein	Carbs	Fat	Fiber	Sodium	Calories

LUNCH	Protein	Carbs	Fat	Fiber	Sodium	Calories

SNACK	Protein	Carbs	Fat	Fiber	Sodium	Calories

DINNER	Protein	Carbs	Fat	Fiber	Sodium	Calories

SNACK	Protein	Carbs	Fat	Fiber	Sodium	Calories
DAILY TOTALS						
DAILY GOALS						
% DAILY GOALS	%	%	%	%	%	%

WATER   1 cup per circle
(1 cup = 8 ounces ~ 240ml)   ○○○○○○○○○○○○○○○○

DATE:		WEEK:		WEIGHT:	

BREAKFAST	Protein	Carbs	Fat	Fiber	Sodium	Calories

SNACK	Protein	Carbs	Fat	Fiber	Sodium	Calories

LUNCH	Protein	Carbs	Fat	Fiber	Sodium	Calories

SNACK	Protein	Carbs	Fat	Fiber	Sodium	Calories

DINNER	Protein	Carbs	Fat	Fiber	Sodium	Calories

SNACK	Protein	Carbs	Fat	Fiber	Sodium	Calories
DAILY TOTALS						
DAILY GOALS						
% DAILY GOALS	%	%	%	%	%	%

WATER   1 cup per circle
(1 cup = 8 ounces ~ 240ml)   ○○○○○○○○○○○○○○○○

DATE:	WEEK:	WEIGHT:

BREAKFAST	Protein	Carbs	Fat	Fiber	Sodium	Calories

SNACK	Protein	Carbs	Fat	Fiber	Sodium	Calories

LUNCH	Protein	Carbs	Fat	Fiber	Sodium	Calories

SNACK	Protein	Carbs	Fat	Fiber	Sodium	Calories

DINNER	Protein	Carbs	Fat	Fiber	Sodium	Calories

SNACK	Protein	Carbs	Fat	Fiber	Sodium	Calories

DAILY TOTALS						
DAILY GOALS						
% DAILY GOALS	%	%	%	%	%	%

WATER   1 cup per circle
(1 cup = 8 ounces ~ 240ml)   ○○○○○○○○○○○○○○○○

DATE:		WEEK:		WEIGHT:		

BREAKFAST	Protein	Carbs	Fat	Fiber	Sodium	Calories

SNACK	Protein	Carbs	Fat	Fiber	Sodium	Calories

LUNCH	Protein	Carbs	Fat	Fiber	Sodium	Calories

SNACK	Protein	Carbs	Fat	Fiber	Sodium	Calories

DINNER	Protein	Carbs	Fat	Fiber	Sodium	Calories

SNACK	Protein	Carbs	Fat	Fiber	Sodium	Calories

DAILY TOTALS						
DAILY GOALS						
% DAILY GOALS	%	%	%	%	%	%

WATER   1 cup per circle
(1 cup = 8 ounces ~ 240ml)   ◯ ◯ ◯ ◯ ◯ ◯ ◯ ◯ ◯ ◯ ◯ ◯ ◯ ◯

| DATE: | | WEEK: | | WEIGHT: | | | |

BREAKFAST	Protein	Carbs	Fat	Fiber	Sodium	Calories

SNACK	Protein	Carbs	Fat	Fiber	Sodium	Calories

LUNCH	Protein	Carbs	Fat	Fiber	Sodium	Calories

SNACK	Protein	Carbs	Fat	Fiber	Sodium	Calories

DINNER	Protein	Carbs	Fat	Fiber	Sodium	Calories

SNACK	Protein	Carbs	Fat	Fiber	Sodium	Calories

DAILY TOTALS						
DAILY GOALS						
% DAILY GOALS	%	%	%	%	%	%

WATER   1 cup per circle
(1 cup = 8 ounces ~ 240ml)   ○○○○○○○○○○○○○○○○○

DATE: [   ]   **WEEK:** [   ]   **WEIGHT:** [   ]

BREAKFAST	Protein	Carbs	Fat	Fiber	Sodium	Calories

SNACK	Protein	Carbs	Fat	Fiber	Sodium	Calories

LUNCH	Protein	Carbs	Fat	Fiber	Sodium	Calories

SNACK	Protein	Carbs	Fat	Fiber	Sodium	Calories

DINNER	Protein	Carbs	Fat	Fiber	Sodium	Calories

SNACK	Protein	Carbs	Fat	Fiber	Sodium	Calories

DAILY TOTALS						
DAILY GOALS						
% DAILY GOALS	%	%	%	%	%	%

WATER   1 cup per circle
(1 cup = 8 ounces ~ 240ml)   ○○○○○○○○○○○○○○○○

DATE:		WEEK:		WEIGHT:	

BREAKFAST	Protein	Carbs	Fat	Fiber	Sodium	Calories

SNACK	Protein	Carbs	Fat	Fiber	Sodium	Calories

LUNCH	Protein	Carbs	Fat	Fiber	Sodium	Calories

SNACK	Protein	Carbs	Fat	Fiber	Sodium	Calories

DINNER	Protein	Carbs	Fat	Fiber	Sodium	Calories

SNACK	Protein	Carbs	Fat	Fiber	Sodium	Calories

DAILY TOTALS						
DAILY GOALS						
% DAILY GOALS	%	%	%	%	%	%

WATER   1 cup per circle
(1 cup = 8 ounces ~ 240ml)   ○○○○○○○○○○○○○○○○○○

DATE:		WEEK:		WEIGHT:	

BREAKFAST	Protein	Carbs	Fat	Fiber	Sodium	Calories

SNACK	Protein	Carbs	Fat	Fiber	Sodium	Calories

LUNCH	Protein	Carbs	Fat	Fiber	Sodium	Calories

SNACK	Protein	Carbs	Fat	Fiber	Sodium	Calories

DINNER	Protein	Carbs	Fat	Fiber	Sodium	Calories

SNACK	Protein	Carbs	Fat	Fiber	Sodium	Calories

DAILY TOTALS						
DAILY GOALS						
% DAILY GOALS	%	%	%	%	%	%

WATER   1 cup per circle
(1 cup = 8 ounces ~ 240ml)   ○○○○○○○○○○○○○○○○

DATE: _____ **WEEK:** _____ **WEIGHT:** _____

BREAKFAST	Protein	Carbs	Fat	Fiber	Sodium	Calories

SNACK	Protein	Carbs	Fat	Fiber	Sodium	Calories

LUNCH	Protein	Carbs	Fat	Fiber	Sodium	Calories

SNACK	Protein	Carbs	Fat	Fiber	Sodium	Calories

DINNER	Protein	Carbs	Fat	Fiber	Sodium	Calories

SNACK	Protein	Carbs	Fat	Fiber	Sodium	Calories

DAILY TOTALS						
DAILY GOALS						
% DAILY GOALS	%	%	%	%	%	%

WATER   1 cup per circle
(1 cup = 8 ounces ~ 240ml)   ○ ○ ○ ○ ○ ○ ○ ○ ○ ○ ○ ○ ○ ○ ○ ○

DATE: [   ]   **WEEK:** [   ]   **WEIGHT:** [   ]

BREAKFAST	Protein	Carbs	Fat	Fiber	Sodium	Calories

SNACK	Protein	Carbs	Fat	Fiber	Sodium	Calories

LUNCH	Protein	Carbs	Fat	Fiber	Sodium	Calories

SNACK	Protein	Carbs	Fat	Fiber	Sodium	Calories

DINNER	Protein	Carbs	Fat	Fiber	Sodium	Calories

SNACK	Protein	Carbs	Fat	Fiber	Sodium	Calories

DAILY TOTALS						
DAILY GOALS						
% DAILY GOALS	%	%	%	%	%	%

WATER   1 cup per circle
(1 cup = 8 ounces ~ 240ml)   ○ ○ ○ ○ ○ ○ ○ ○ ○ ○ ○ ○ ○ ○ ○

DATE: _____ **WEEK:** _____ **WEIGHT:** _____

BREAKFAST	Protein	Carbs	Fat	Fiber	Sodium	Calories

SNACK	Protein	Carbs	Fat	Fiber	Sodium	Calories

LUNCH	Protein	Carbs	Fat	Fiber	Sodium	Calories

SNACK	Protein	Carbs	Fat	Fiber	Sodium	Calories

DINNER	Protein	Carbs	Fat	Fiber	Sodium	Calories

SNACK	Protein	Carbs	Fat	Fiber	Sodium	Calories

DAILY TOTALS						
DAILY GOALS						
% DAILY GOALS	%	%	%	%	%	%

WATER   1 cup per circle
(1 cup = 8 ounces ~ 240ml)   ○○○○○○○○○○○○○○○○

DATE:	WEEK:	WEIGHT:

BREAKFAST	Protein	Carbs	Fat	Fiber	Sodium	Calories

SNACK	Protein	Carbs	Fat	Fiber	Sodium	Calories

LUNCH	Protein	Carbs	Fat	Fiber	Sodium	Calories

SNACK	Protein	Carbs	Fat	Fiber	Sodium	Calories

DINNER	Protein	Carbs	Fat	Fiber	Sodium	Calories

SNACK	Protein	Carbs	Fat	Fiber	Sodium	Calories

DAILY TOTALS						
DAILY GOALS						
% DAILY GOALS	%	%	%	%	%	%

WATER   1 cup per circle
(1 cup = 8 ounces ~ 240ml)   ○○○○○○○○○○○○○○○○

DATE:		WEEK:		WEIGHT:		

BREAKFAST	Protein	Carbs	Fat	Fiber	Sodium	Calories

SNACK	Protein	Carbs	Fat	Fiber	Sodium	Calories

LUNCH	Protein	Carbs	Fat	Fiber	Sodium	Calories

SNACK	Protein	Carbs	Fat	Fiber	Sodium	Calories

DINNER	Protein	Carbs	Fat	Fiber	Sodium	Calories

SNACK	Protein	Carbs	Fat	Fiber	Sodium	Calories

DAILY TOTALS						
DAILY GOALS						
% DAILY GOALS	%	%	%	%	%	%

WATER   1 cup per circle
(1 cup = 8 ounces ~ 240ml)   ○○○○○○○○○○○○○○○○○

DATE:	WEEK:	WEIGHT:

BREAKFAST	Protein	Carbs	Fat	Fiber	Sodium	Calories

SNACK	Protein	Carbs	Fat	Fiber	Sodium	Calories

LUNCH	Protein	Carbs	Fat	Fiber	Sodium	Calories

SNACK	Protein	Carbs	Fat	Fiber	Sodium	Calories

DINNER	Protein	Carbs	Fat	Fiber	Sodium	Calories

SNACK	Protein	Carbs	Fat	Fiber	Sodium	Calories

DAILY TOTALS						
DAILY GOALS						
% DAILY GOALS	%	%	%	%	%	%

WATER   1 cup per circle
(1 cup = 8 ounces ~ 240ml)   ○○○○○○○○○○○○○○○

DATE: _____ **WEEK:** _____ **WEIGHT:** _____

BREAKFAST	Protein	Carbs	Fat	Fiber	Sodium	Calories

SNACK	Protein	Carbs	Fat	Fiber	Sodium	Calories

LUNCH	Protein	Carbs	Fat	Fiber	Sodium	Calories

SNACK	Protein	Carbs	Fat	Fiber	Sodium	Calories

DINNER	Protein	Carbs	Fat	Fiber	Sodium	Calories

SNACK	Protein	Carbs	Fat	Fiber	Sodium	Calories

	Protein	Carbs	Fat	Fiber	Sodium	Calories
DAILY TOTALS						
DAILY GOALS						
% DAILY GOALS	%	%	%	%	%	%

WATER   1 cup per circle
(1 cup = 8 ounces ~ 240ml)   ○ ○ ○ ○ ○ ○ ○ ○ ○ ○ ○ ○ ○ ○ ○ ○

DATE: _____   WEEK: _____   WEIGHT: _____

BREAKFAST	Protein	Carbs	Fat	Fiber	Sodium	Calories

SNACK	Protein	Carbs	Fat	Fiber	Sodium	Calories

LUNCH	Protein	Carbs	Fat	Fiber	Sodium	Calories

SNACK	Protein	Carbs	Fat	Fiber	Sodium	Calories

DINNER	Protein	Carbs	Fat	Fiber	Sodium	Calories

SNACK	Protein	Carbs	Fat	Fiber	Sodium	Calories

	Protein	Carbs	Fat	Fiber	Sodium	Calories
DAILY TOTALS						
DAILY GOALS						
% DAILY GOALS	%	%	%	%	%	%

WATER 1 cup per circle
(1 cup = 8 ounces ~ 240ml)   ○○○○○○○○○○○○○○○

DATE:		WEEK:		WEIGHT:			

BREAKFAST	Protein	Carbs	Fat	Fiber	Sodium	Calories

SNACK	Protein	Carbs	Fat	Fiber	Sodium	Calories

LUNCH	Protein	Carbs	Fat	Fiber	Sodium	Calories

SNACK	Protein	Carbs	Fat	Fiber	Sodium	Calories

DINNER	Protein	Carbs	Fat	Fiber	Sodium	Calories

SNACK	Protein	Carbs	Fat	Fiber	Sodium	Calories

DAILY TOTALS						
DAILY GOALS						
% DAILY GOALS	%	%	%	%	%	%

WATER   1 cup per circle
(1 cup = 8 ounces ~ 240ml)   ○ ○ ○ ○ ○ ○ ○ ○ ○ ○ ○ ○ ○ ○ ○ ○

DATE:	WEEK:	WEIGHT:

BREAKFAST	Protein	Carbs	Fat	Fiber	Sodium	Calories

SNACK	Protein	Carbs	Fat	Fiber	Sodium	Calories

LUNCH	Protein	Carbs	Fat	Fiber	Sodium	Calories

SNACK	Protein	Carbs	Fat	Fiber	Sodium	Calories

DINNER	Protein	Carbs	Fat	Fiber	Sodium	Calories

SNACK	Protein	Carbs	Fat	Fiber	Sodium	Calories

DAILY TOTALS						
DAILY GOALS						
% DAILY GOALS	%	%	%	%	%	%

WATER   1 cup per circle
(1 cup = 8 ounces ~ 240ml)   ○○○○○○○○○○○○○○○○

DATE:		WEEK:		WEIGHT:	

BREAKFAST	Protein	Carbs	Fat	Fiber	Sodium	Calories

SNACK	Protein	Carbs	Fat	Fiber	Sodium	Calories

LUNCH	Protein	Carbs	Fat	Fiber	Sodium	Calories

SNACK	Protein	Carbs	Fat	Fiber	Sodium	Calories

DINNER	Protein	Carbs	Fat	Fiber	Sodium	Calories

SNACK	Protein	Carbs	Fat	Fiber	Sodium	Calories

DAILY TOTALS						
DAILY GOALS						
% DAILY GOALS	%	%	%	%	%	%

WATER   1 cup per circle
(1 cup = 8 ounces ~ 240ml)   ○○○○○○○○○○○○○○○○

DATE:		WEEK:		WEIGHT:	

BREAKFAST	Protein	Carbs	Fat	Fiber	Sodium	Calories

SNACK	Protein	Carbs	Fat	Fiber	Sodium	Calories

LUNCH	Protein	Carbs	Fat	Fiber	Sodium	Calories

SNACK	Protein	Carbs	Fat	Fiber	Sodium	Calories

DINNER	Protein	Carbs	Fat	Fiber	Sodium	Calories

SNACK	Protein	Carbs	Fat	Fiber	Sodium	Calories

	Protein	Carbs	Fat	Fiber	Sodium	Calories
DAILY TOTALS						
DAILY GOALS						
% DAILY GOALS	%	%	%	%	%	%

WATER   1 cup per circle
(1 cup = 8 ounces ~ 240ml)   ○○○○○○○○○○○○○○○

DATE:	WEEK:	WEIGHT:

BREAKFAST	Protein	Carbs	Fat	Fiber	Sodium	Calories

SNACK	Protein	Carbs	Fat	Fiber	Sodium	Calories

LUNCH	Protein	Carbs	Fat	Fiber	Sodium	Calories

SNACK	Protein	Carbs	Fat	Fiber	Sodium	Calories

DINNER	Protein	Carbs	Fat	Fiber	Sodium	Calories

SNACK	Protein	Carbs	Fat	Fiber	Sodium	Calories

DAILY TOTALS						
DAILY GOALS						
% DAILY GOALS	%	%	%	%	%	%

WATER   1 cup per circle
(1 cup = 8 ounces ~ 240ml)   ○ ○ ○ ○ ○ ○ ○ ○ ○ ○ ○ ○ ○ ○ ○ ○

DATE: [   ]   WEEK: [   ]   WEIGHT: [   ]

BREAKFAST	Protein	Carbs	Fat	Fiber	Sodium	Calories

SNACK	Protein	Carbs	Fat	Fiber	Sodium	Calories

LUNCH	Protein	Carbs	Fat	Fiber	Sodium	Calories

SNACK	Protein	Carbs	Fat	Fiber	Sodium	Calories

DINNER	Protein	Carbs	Fat	Fiber	Sodium	Calories

SNACK	Protein	Carbs	Fat	Fiber	Sodium	Calories

DAILY TOTALS						
DAILY GOALS						
% DAILY GOALS	%	%	%	%	%	%

WATER   1 cup per circle
(1 cup = 8 ounces ~ 240ml)   ○○○○○○○○○○○○○○○○○

DATE:	WEEK:	WEIGHT:

BREAKFAST	Protein	Carbs	Fat	Fiber	Sodium	Calories

SNACK	Protein	Carbs	Fat	Fiber	Sodium	Calories

LUNCH	Protein	Carbs	Fat	Fiber	Sodium	Calories

SNACK	Protein	Carbs	Fat	Fiber	Sodium	Calories

DINNER	Protein	Carbs	Fat	Fiber	Sodium	Calories

SNACK	Protein	Carbs	Fat	Fiber	Sodium	Calories

DAILY TOTALS						
DAILY GOALS						
% DAILY GOALS	%	%	%	%	%	%

WATER   1 cup per circle
(1 cup = 8 ounces ~ 240ml)   ○ ○ ○ ○ ○ ○ ○ ○ ○ ○ ○ ○ ○ ○ ○ ○

DATE: [   ]   WEEK: [   ]   WEIGHT: [   ]

BREAKFAST	Protein	Carbs	Fat	Fiber	Sodium	Calories

SNACK	Protein	Carbs	Fat	Fiber	Sodium	Calories

LUNCH	Protein	Carbs	Fat	Fiber	Sodium	Calories

SNACK	Protein	Carbs	Fat	Fiber	Sodium	Calories

DINNER	Protein	Carbs	Fat	Fiber	Sodium	Calories

SNACK	Protein	Carbs	Fat	Fiber	Sodium	Calories

DAILY TOTALS						
DAILY GOALS						
% DAILY GOALS	%	%	%	%	%	%

WATER   1 cup per circle
(1 cup = 8 ounces ~ 240ml)   ○○○○○○○○○○○○○○○○

DATE:	WEEK:	WEIGHT:

BREAKFAST	Protein	Carbs	Fat	Fiber	Sodium	Calories

SNACK	Protein	Carbs	Fat	Fiber	Sodium	Calories

LUNCH	Protein	Carbs	Fat	Fiber	Sodium	Calories

SNACK	Protein	Carbs	Fat	Fiber	Sodium	Calories

DINNER	Protein	Carbs	Fat	Fiber	Sodium	Calories

SNACK	Protein	Carbs	Fat	Fiber	Sodium	Calories

DAILY TOTALS						
DAILY GOALS						
% DAILY GOALS	%	%	%	%	%	%

WATER 1 cup per circle
(1 cup = 8 ounces ~ 240ml)   ○○○○○○○○○○○○○○○○

DATE:	WEEK:	WEIGHT:

BREAKFAST	Protein	Carbs	Fat	Fiber	Sodium	Calories

SNACK	Protein	Carbs	Fat	Fiber	Sodium	Calories

LUNCH	Protein	Carbs	Fat	Fiber	Sodium	Calories

SNACK	Protein	Carbs	Fat	Fiber	Sodium	Calories

DINNER	Protein	Carbs	Fat	Fiber	Sodium	Calories

SNACK	Protein	Carbs	Fat	Fiber	Sodium	Calories

DAILY TOTALS						
DAILY GOALS						
% DAILY GOALS	%	%	%	%	%	%

WATER   1 cup per circle
(1 cup = 8 ounces ~ 240ml)   ○○○○○○○○○○○○○○○○

DATE:	WEEK:	WEIGHT:

BREAKFAST	Protein	Carbs	Fat	Fiber	Sodium	Calories

SNACK	Protein	Carbs	Fat	Fiber	Sodium	Calories

LUNCH	Protein	Carbs	Fat	Fiber	Sodium	Calories

SNACK	Protein	Carbs	Fat	Fiber	Sodium	Calories

DINNER	Protein	Carbs	Fat	Fiber	Sodium	Calories

SNACK	Protein	Carbs	Fat	Fiber	Sodium	Calories

DAILY TOTALS						
DAILY GOALS						
% DAILY GOALS	%	%	%	%	%	%

WATER   1 cup per circle
(1 cup = 8 ounces ~ 240ml)   ○○○○○○○○○○○○○○○○○

DATE: _____ **WEEK:** _____ **WEIGHT:** _____

BREAKFAST	Protein	Carbs	Fat	Fiber	Sodium	Calories

SNACK	Protein	Carbs	Fat	Fiber	Sodium	Calories

LUNCH	Protein	Carbs	Fat	Fiber	Sodium	Calories

SNACK	Protein	Carbs	Fat	Fiber	Sodium	Calories

DINNER	Protein	Carbs	Fat	Fiber	Sodium	Calories

SNACK	Protein	Carbs	Fat	Fiber	Sodium	Calories

	Protein	Carbs	Fat	Fiber	Sodium	Calories
DAILY TOTALS						
DAILY GOALS						
% DAILY GOALS	%	%	%	%	%	%

WATER   1 cup per circle
(1 cup = 8 ounces ~ 240ml)   ○○○○○○○○○○○○○○○○○

DATE:	WEEK:	WEIGHT:

BREAKFAST	Protein	Carbs	Fat	Fiber	Sodium	Calories

SNACK	Protein	Carbs	Fat	Fiber	Sodium	Calories

LUNCH	Protein	Carbs	Fat	Fiber	Sodium	Calories

SNACK	Protein	Carbs	Fat	Fiber	Sodium	Calories

DINNER	Protein	Carbs	Fat	Fiber	Sodium	Calories

SNACK	Protein	Carbs	Fat	Fiber	Sodium	Calories

DAILY TOTALS						
DAILY GOALS						
% DAILY GOALS	%	%	%	%	%	%

WATER   1 cup per circle
(1 cup = 8 ounces ~ 240ml)   ○○○○○○○○○○○○○○○○

DATE:		WEEK:		WEIGHT:	

BREAKFAST	Protein	Carbs	Fat	Fiber	Sodium	Calories

SNACK	Protein	Carbs	Fat	Fiber	Sodium	Calories

LUNCH	Protein	Carbs	Fat	Fiber	Sodium	Calories

SNACK	Protein	Carbs	Fat	Fiber	Sodium	Calories

DINNER	Protein	Carbs	Fat	Fiber	Sodium	Calories

SNACK	Protein	Carbs	Fat	Fiber	Sodium	Calories

DAILY TOTALS						
DAILY GOALS						
% DAILY GOALS	%	%	%	%	%	%

WATER   1 cup per circle
(1 cup = 8 ounces ~ 240ml)   ○○○○○○○○○○○○○○○

DATE:	WEEK:	WEIGHT:

BREAKFAST	Protein	Carbs	Fat	Fiber	Sodium	Calories

SNACK	Protein	Carbs	Fat	Fiber	Sodium	Calories

LUNCH	Protein	Carbs	Fat	Fiber	Sodium	Calories

SNACK	Protein	Carbs	Fat	Fiber	Sodium	Calories

DINNER	Protein	Carbs	Fat	Fiber	Sodium	Calories

SNACK	Protein	Carbs	Fat	Fiber	Sodium	Calories

DAILY TOTALS						
DAILY GOALS						
% DAILY GOALS	%	%	%	%	%	%

WATER   1 cup per circle
(1 cup = 8 ounces ~ 240ml)   ○○○○○○○○○○○○○○○○○○

DATE:		WEEK:		WEIGHT:	

BREAKFAST	Protein	Carbs	Fat	Fiber	Sodium	Calories

SNACK	Protein	Carbs	Fat	Fiber	Sodium	Calories

LUNCH	Protein	Carbs	Fat	Fiber	Sodium	Calories

SNACK	Protein	Carbs	Fat	Fiber	Sodium	Calories

DINNER	Protein	Carbs	Fat	Fiber	Sodium	Calories

SNACK	Protein	Carbs	Fat	Fiber	Sodium	Calories
DAILY TOTALS						
DAILY GOALS						
% DAILY GOALS	%	%	%	%	%	%

WATER   1 cup per circle
(1 cup = 8 ounces ~ 240ml)   ○○○○○○○○○○○○○○○

DATE:	WEEK:	WEIGHT:

BREAKFAST	Protein	Carbs	Fat	Fiber	Sodium	Calories

SNACK	Protein	Carbs	Fat	Fiber	Sodium	Calories

LUNCH	Protein	Carbs	Fat	Fiber	Sodium	Calories

SNACK	Protein	Carbs	Fat	Fiber	Sodium	Calories

DINNER	Protein	Carbs	Fat	Fiber	Sodium	Calories

SNACK	Protein	Carbs	Fat	Fiber	Sodium	Calories

DAILY TOTALS						
DAILY GOALS						
% DAILY GOALS	%	%	%	%	%	%

WATER   1 cup per circle
(1 cup = 8 ounces ~ 240ml)   ○ ○ ○ ○ ○ ○ ○ ○ ○ ○ ○ ○ ○ ○ ○ ○

DATE:		WEEK:		WEIGHT:			

BREAKFAST	Protein	Carbs	Fat	Fiber	Sodium	Calories

SNACK	Protein	Carbs	Fat	Fiber	Sodium	Calories

LUNCH	Protein	Carbs	Fat	Fiber	Sodium	Calories

SNACK	Protein	Carbs	Fat	Fiber	Sodium	Calories

DINNER	Protein	Carbs	Fat	Fiber	Sodium	Calories

SNACK	Protein	Carbs	Fat	Fiber	Sodium	Calories

DAILY TOTALS						
DAILY GOALS						
% DAILY GOALS	%	%	%	%	%	%

WATER   1 cup per circle
(1 cup = 8 ounces ~ 240ml)   ○○○○○○○○○○○○○○○○

DATE:	WEEK:	WEIGHT:

BREAKFAST	Protein	Carbs	Fat	Fiber	Sodium	Calories

SNACK	Protein	Carbs	Fat	Fiber	Sodium	Calories

LUNCH	Protein	Carbs	Fat	Fiber	Sodium	Calories

SNACK	Protein	Carbs	Fat	Fiber	Sodium	Calories

DINNER	Protein	Carbs	Fat	Fiber	Sodium	Calories

SNACK	Protein	Carbs	Fat	Fiber	Sodium	Calories
DAILY TOTALS						
DAILY GOALS						
% DAILY GOALS	%	%	%	%	%	%

WATER   1 cup per circle
(1 cup = 8 ounces ~ 240ml)   ○○○○○○○○○○○○○○○○○○

DATE: **WEEK:**   **WEIGHT:**

BREAKFAST	Protein	Carbs	Fat	Fiber	Sodium	Calories
SNACK	Protein	Carbs	Fat	Fiber	Sodium	Calories
LUNCH	Protein	Carbs	Fat	Fiber	Sodium	Calories
SNACK	Protein	Carbs	Fat	Fiber	Sodium	Calories
DINNER	Protein	Carbs	Fat	Fiber	Sodium	Calories
SNACK	Protein	Carbs	Fat	Fiber	Sodium	Calories
DAILY TOTALS						
DAILY GOALS						
% DAILY GOALS	%	%	%	%	%	%

WATER   1 cup per circle
(1 cup = 8 ounces ~ 240ml)   ○○○○○○○○○○○○○○○

DATE:	WEEK:	WEIGHT:

BREAKFAST	Protein	Carbs	Fat	Fiber	Sodium	Calories

SNACK	Protein	Carbs	Fat	Fiber	Sodium	Calories

LUNCH	Protein	Carbs	Fat	Fiber	Sodium	Calories

SNACK	Protein	Carbs	Fat	Fiber	Sodium	Calories

DINNER	Protein	Carbs	Fat	Fiber	Sodium	Calories

SNACK	Protein	Carbs	Fat	Fiber	Sodium	Calories

DAILY TOTALS						
DAILY GOALS						
% DAILY GOALS	%	%	%	%	%	%

WATER   1 cup per circle
(1 cup = 8 ounces ~ 240ml)   ○ ○ ○ ○ ○ ○ ○ ○ ○ ○ ○ ○ ○ ○ ○

DATE:		WEEK:		WEIGHT:	

BREAKFAST	Protein	Carbs	Fat	Fiber	Sodium	Calories

SNACK	Protein	Carbs	Fat	Fiber	Sodium	Calories

LUNCH	Protein	Carbs	Fat	Fiber	Sodium	Calories

SNACK	Protein	Carbs	Fat	Fiber	Sodium	Calories

DINNER	Protein	Carbs	Fat	Fiber	Sodium	Calories

SNACK	Protein	Carbs	Fat	Fiber	Sodium	Calories
DAILY TOTALS						
DAILY GOALS						
% DAILY GOALS	%	%	%	%	%	%

WATER 1 cup per circle
(1 cup = 8 ounces ~ 240ml) ○○○○○○○○○○○○○○○○

DATE: _____ **WEEK:** _____ **WEIGHT:** _____

BREAKFAST	Protein	Carbs	Fat	Fiber	Sodium	Calories

SNACK	Protein	Carbs	Fat	Fiber	Sodium	Calories

LUNCH	Protein	Carbs	Fat	Fiber	Sodium	Calories

SNACK	Protein	Carbs	Fat	Fiber	Sodium	Calories

DINNER	Protein	Carbs	Fat	Fiber	Sodium	Calories

SNACK	Protein	Carbs	Fat	Fiber	Sodium	Calories

DAILY TOTALS						
DAILY GOALS						
% DAILY GOALS	%	%	%	%	%	%

WATER   1 cup per circle
(1 cup = 8 ounces ~ 240ml)   ○○○○○○○○○○○○○○○○

DATE: _____ WEEK: _____ WEIGHT: _____

BREAKFAST	Protein	Carbs	Fat	Fiber	Sodium	Calories

SNACK	Protein	Carbs	Fat	Fiber	Sodium	Calories

LUNCH	Protein	Carbs	Fat	Fiber	Sodium	Calories

SNACK	Protein	Carbs	Fat	Fiber	Sodium	Calories

DINNER	Protein	Carbs	Fat	Fiber	Sodium	Calories

SNACK	Protein	Carbs	Fat	Fiber	Sodium	Calories
DAILY TOTALS						
DAILY GOALS						
% DAILY GOALS	%	%	%	%	%	%

WATER   1 cup per circle
(1 cup = 8 ounces ~ 240ml)   ○○○○○○○○○○○○○○○

DATE:		WEEK:		WEIGHT:		

BREAKFAST	Protein	Carbs	Fat	Fiber	Sodium	Calories

SNACK	Protein	Carbs	Fat	Fiber	Sodium	Calories

LUNCH	Protein	Carbs	Fat	Fiber	Sodium	Calories

SNACK	Protein	Carbs	Fat	Fiber	Sodium	Calories

DINNER	Protein	Carbs	Fat	Fiber	Sodium	Calories

SNACK	Protein	Carbs	Fat	Fiber	Sodium	Calories

DAILY TOTALS						
DAILY GOALS						
% DAILY GOALS	%	%	%	%	%	%

WATER   1 cup per circle
(1 cup = 8 ounces ~ 240ml)   ○○○○○○○○○○○○○○○○○

DATE: | **WEEK:** | **WEIGHT:**

BREAKFAST	Protein	Carbs	Fat	Fiber	Sodium	Calories

SNACK	Protein	Carbs	Fat	Fiber	Sodium	Calories

LUNCH	Protein	Carbs	Fat	Fiber	Sodium	Calories

SNACK	Protein	Carbs	Fat	Fiber	Sodium	Calories

DINNER	Protein	Carbs	Fat	Fiber	Sodium	Calories

SNACK	Protein	Carbs	Fat	Fiber	Sodium	Calories

DAILY TOTALS						
DAILY GOALS						
% DAILY GOALS	%	%	%	%	%	%

WATER 1 cup per circle
(1 cup = 8 ounces ~ 240ml) ○○○○○○○○○○○○○○○○

DATE: [   ] **WEEK:** [   ] **WEIGHT:** [   ]

BREAKFAST	Protein	Carbs	Fat	Fiber	Sodium	Calories

SNACK	Protein	Carbs	Fat	Fiber	Sodium	Calories

LUNCH	Protein	Carbs	Fat	Fiber	Sodium	Calories

SNACK	Protein	Carbs	Fat	Fiber	Sodium	Calories

DINNER	Protein	Carbs	Fat	Fiber	Sodium	Calories

SNACK	Protein	Carbs	Fat	Fiber	Sodium	Calories

	Protein	Carbs	Fat	Fiber	Sodium	Calories
DAILY TOTALS						
DAILY GOALS						
% DAILY GOALS	%	%	%	%	%	%

WATER 1 cup per circle
(1 cup = 8 ounces ~ 240ml)   ○○○○○○○○○○○○○○○○

DATE:	WEEK:	WEIGHT:

BREAKFAST	Protein	Carbs	Fat	Fiber	Sodium	Calories

SNACK	Protein	Carbs	Fat	Fiber	Sodium	Calories

LUNCH	Protein	Carbs	Fat	Fiber	Sodium	Calories

SNACK	Protein	Carbs	Fat	Fiber	Sodium	Calories

DINNER	Protein	Carbs	Fat	Fiber	Sodium	Calories

SNACK	Protein	Carbs	Fat	Fiber	Sodium	Calories

DAILY TOTALS						
DAILY GOALS						
% DAILY GOALS	%	%	%	%	%	%

WATER   1 cup per circle
(1 cup = 8 ounces ~ 240ml)   ○○○○○○○○○○○○○○○○

DATE:	WEEK:	WEIGHT:

BREAKFAST	Protein	Carbs	Fat	Fiber	Sodium	Calories

SNACK	Protein	Carbs	Fat	Fiber	Sodium	Calories

LUNCH	Protein	Carbs	Fat	Fiber	Sodium	Calories

SNACK	Protein	Carbs	Fat	Fiber	Sodium	Calories

DINNER	Protein	Carbs	Fat	Fiber	Sodium	Calories

SNACK	Protein	Carbs	Fat	Fiber	Sodium	Calories

DAILY TOTALS						
DAILY GOALS						
% DAILY GOALS	%	%	%	%	%	%

WATER   1 cup per circle
(1 cup = 8 ounces ~ 240ml)   ○ ○ ○ ○ ○ ○ ○ ○ ○ ○ ○ ○ ○ ○ ○ ○

DATE: | **WEEK:** | **WEIGHT:**

BREAKFAST	Protein	Carbs	Fat	Fiber	Sodium	Calories

SNACK	Protein	Carbs	Fat	Fiber	Sodium	Calories

LUNCH	Protein	Carbs	Fat	Fiber	Sodium	Calories

SNACK	Protein	Carbs	Fat	Fiber	Sodium	Calories

DINNER	Protein	Carbs	Fat	Fiber	Sodium	Calories

SNACK	Protein	Carbs	Fat	Fiber	Sodium	Calories

DAILY TOTALS						
DAILY GOALS						
% DAILY GOALS	%	%	%	%	%	%

WATER   1 cup per circle
(1 cup = 8 ounces ~ 240ml)   ○ ○ ○ ○ ○ ○ ○ ○ ○ ○ ○ ○ ○ ○ ○ ○

DATE:		WEEK:		WEIGHT:	

BREAKFAST	Protein	Carbs	Fat	Fiber	Sodium	Calories

SNACK	Protein	Carbs	Fat	Fiber	Sodium	Calories

LUNCH	Protein	Carbs	Fat	Fiber	Sodium	Calories

SNACK	Protein	Carbs	Fat	Fiber	Sodium	Calories

DINNER	Protein	Carbs	Fat	Fiber	Sodium	Calories

SNACK	Protein	Carbs	Fat	Fiber	Sodium	Calories

DAILY TOTALS						
DAILY GOALS						
% DAILY GOALS	%	%	%	%	%	%

WATER   1 cup per circle
(1 cup = 8 ounces ~ 240ml)   ○○○○○○○○○○○○○○○○○

DATE: _____ WEEK: _____ WEIGHT: _____

BREAKFAST	Protein	Carbs	Fat	Fiber	Sodium	Calories

SNACK	Protein	Carbs	Fat	Fiber	Sodium	Calories

LUNCH	Protein	Carbs	Fat	Fiber	Sodium	Calories

SNACK	Protein	Carbs	Fat	Fiber	Sodium	Calories

DINNER	Protein	Carbs	Fat	Fiber	Sodium	Calories

SNACK	Protein	Carbs	Fat	Fiber	Sodium	Calories

DAILY TOTALS						
DAILY GOALS						
% DAILY GOALS	%	%	%	%	%	%

WATER   1 cup per circle
(1 cup = 8 ounces ~ 240ml)   ○○○○○○○○○○○○○○○○

Printed in Great Britain
by Amazon

35832875R00068